HERBS FOR ARTHRITIS FLARE UPS

Empower Your Healing Journey: Harnessing The Power Of Natural Remedies With Holistic Approaches

DR. JEREMY ALLEY

Disclaimer:

The information provided in this book, is intended for general informational purposes only and should not be considered as professional advice.

The author has made every effort to ensure the accuracy of the information presented. However, readers are advised to consult with a qualified healthcare professional before attempting any herbal remedies or making significant changes to their wellness routine. Individual health conditions vary, and what may be suitable for one person may not be appropriate for another.

It is important to note that the author is not in any endorsement deal, partnership, or affiliation with any organization, brand, or company mentioned in this book. Any references to specific products or services are based on the author's personal experience or general knowledge and do not imply an endorsement or promotion of those products or services.

Contents

Overview

A common and crippling illness that affects millions of individuals worldwide is arthritis. The discomfort, swelling, and rigidity brought on by arthritis can have a serious negative effect on a person's quality of life. Even while doctors frequently prescribe drugs and physical therapy as treatments, many people look for other ways to manage their symptoms. For some people with arthritis, herbal medicines have shown to be a source of relief, providing a holistic and natural approach to managing the difficulties presented by flare-ups.

An Overview of Arthritis

A collection of disorders collectively referred to as arthritis is defined by inflammation of the joints, resulting in pain, edema, and reduced range of motion. Rheumatoid arthritis and osteoarthritis are the two most prevalent forms of arthritis. Rheumatoid arthritis is characterized by the immune system attacking the joints, whereas osteoarthritis is mostly related to the deterioration of joint cartilage. Whatever the precise kind, arthritis can lead to flare-ups, which are periods when the symptoms worsen and become more difficult to control.

Investigating efficient therapy options for arthritis requires an understanding of its fundamental mechanics. An important factor in the development of arthritis is inflammation, which also contributes to joint pain and damage. The goals of conventional therapy are frequent symptom relief and disease progression. Herbal treatments, on the other hand, provide a supplementary strategy by reducing inflammation and offering relief without the possible adverse effects of some drugs.

The Value of Herbal Treatments

There are various reasons why using herbal treatments to treat arthritic flare-ups is becoming more and more common. The comparatively decreased risk of side effects in comparison to pharmaceutical therapies is one important benefit. Traditional medical systems have been using several herbal medicines for decades, and their safety profiles are well-established. Herbal treatments also frequently provide a comprehensive approach to health, treating symptoms as well as enhancing general well-being.

Because they have analgesic and anti-inflammatory qualities, herbs are useful tools for treating the symptoms of arthritis. Certain herbs can reduce the autoimmune response associated with illnesses like rheumatoid arthritis by helping to control the immune system. Herbal therapies are holistic in that they take into account lifestyle aspects as well, stressing the importance of food modifications, exercise, and stress management in managing arthritis.

Herbal medicines are an effective way to manage flare-ups of arthritis, as more people look for sustainable and natural ways to health. The ensuing segments will delve into certain herbs and herbal combinations that exhibit the potential to mitigate the symptoms linked to arthritis, providing a comprehensive and integrated strategy to enhance the well-being of individuals impacted by this ailment.

CHAPTER ONE

RECOGNIZING ARTHRITIS

The frequent and crippling disorder known as arthritis is characterized by inflammation of the joints, which results in pain, stiffness, and decreased movement.

To properly manage and relieve the symptoms of arthritis, it is imperative to comprehend its numerous elements.

Types Of Arthritis

Arthritis comes in a variety of forms, each with distinct traits and underlying reasons. The most common types include gout, psoriatic arthritis, rheumatoid arthritis, and osteoarthritis.

Determining the best herbal treatments for arthritis symptoms requires an understanding of the particular form of arthritis.

Reasons And Initiators

A person's lifestyle, surroundings, and genetic makeup can all contribute to the development of arthritis. Obesity, joint traumas, and aging are common factors in the development of arthritis. Furthermore, autoimmune reactions contribute to several forms of arthritis, including rheumatoid arthritis. For a herbal cure to be effective, it is essential to determine the reasons and triggers of arthritis.

Signs And Prognosis

For early diagnosis and management of arthritis, it is essential to recognize its signs. Joint discomfort, edema, stiffness, and a reduction in range of motion are typical symptoms. A complete examination, a review of medical history, and imaging tests like MRIs or X-rays are frequently used in the diagnosis process. Tailoring herbal treatments to treat flare-ups of arthritis requires an understanding of the symptoms and a proper diagnosis.

Herbal Treatments For Flare-Up Arthritis

For generations, people with arthritis have used herbal medicines to control their symptoms and reduce flare-ups. More often than not, these natural substitutes for prescription drugs provide relief with fewer adverse effects. To properly manage flare-ups of arthritis, it is vital to investigate and comprehend the many herbal possibilities.

Curcumin And Turmeric

Curcumin, a strong anti-inflammatory molecule, is found in turmeric, a spice that is frequently used in Indian cooking. Curcumin may lessen inflammation brought on by arthritis and ease pain, according to research. Adding turmeric to food or supplementing with curcumin may help control flare-ups of arthritis.

Ginger

Another herb with anti-inflammatory qualities is ginger. Gingerol, a bioactive substance with possible analgesic properties, is present in it. During flare-ups, taking ginger pills, making ginger tea, or adding fresh ginger to meals may help lessen the discomfort associated with arthritis.

Boswellia

Boswellia extract, which is made from the resin of the Boswellia tree, has anti-inflammatory qualities that may help people with arthritis. According to studies, boswellia is a promising herbal treatment for arthritic flare-ups since it may aid with pain reduction and joint function improvement.

Verdant Tea

Polyphenols, found in abundance in green tea, have anti-inflammatory and antioxidant qualities.

These substances might lessen the symptoms of arthritis.

Regularly consuming green tea or taking green tea supplements may help to lower inflammation and relieve pain when arthritis flares up.

Willow Bark

Salicin, a naturally occurring substance with anti-inflammatory and pain-relieving qualities, is found in willow bark.

 It is regarded as an all-natural substitute for aspirin. Supplements of willow bark extract may be useful in treating pain and discomfort associated with flare-ups of arthritis.

In comparison to conventional pharmaceuticals, herbal therapies provide a more comprehensive approach to managing arthritic flare-ups by relieving symptoms and possibly minimizing adverse effects.

To guarantee safety and efficacy, you should speak with a healthcare provider before implementing herbal treatments into your arthritis treatment strategy. Knowing the range of options available can enable people to make well-informed decisions while managing the difficulties associated with arthritis.

CHAPTER TWO

HERBS TO RELIEVE ARTHRITIS

Joint inflammation is the hallmark of arthritis, a disorder that frequently causes pain and discomfort. Even while there are traditional therapies for arthritis, many people look for complementary methods, such as using herbal medicines, to control their symptoms. In this investigation of herbal remedies, we examine several herbs well-known for their capacity to alleviate flare-ups of arthritis.

Nature's Anti-Inflammatory Spice: Turmeric

The bright yellow spice turmeric comes from the Curcuma longa plant, and it's well known for its strong anti-inflammatory qualities. Turmeric's key ingredient, curcumin, is well-liked by people with arthritic symptoms since research has shown that it can lower inflammation in the body. There are several ways to eat turmeric, including as a supplement, in teas, and curries.

Ginger: Relieving Arthritis

Ginger is another highly respected herb in the field of arthritis therapy. Due to its anti-inflammatory and analgesic qualities, ginger can help reduce arthritis-related joint discomfort. Teas, infusions, and cooking spice are some ways to include it in your diet. Some people can get comfort by directly using topical treatments loaded with ginger on their afflicted joints.

Natural Anti-Arthritic: Boswellia

The anti-arthritic qualities of Boswellia, which are made from the resin of Boswellia serrata trees, are well known. Boswellic acids, the main ingredients in boswellia, have been investigated for their ability to lower inflammation and suppress the inflammatory reaction linked to some forms of arthritis. There are

Boswellia supplements that make it easy to use this plant in an arthritis treatment plan.

Devil's Claw: Reducing Unease

The South African native plant known as "devil's claw" has long been used in traditional medicine to treat a variety of conditions, including arthritis. The plant known as Devil's Claw has anti-inflammatory chemicals in its root, which could explain why it can help relieve arthritic pain. You can consume Devil's Claw as tinctures, teas, or pills.

Wiltshire Bark: The Natural Aspirin

Willow bark is a natural pain and inflammation reliever that has been used for ages. It is derived from the bark of the willow tree. Willow bark has a substance called salicin, which has analgesic and anti-inflammatory properties, much like aspirin. Those looking for a more gentle option for treating their arthritis symptoms naturally may want to consider willow bark teas or supplements.

Additional Herbal Supporters

In addition to the herbs indicated above, there are a few other herbal companions that can help relieve arthritis. These include aloe vera, which is well recognized for its calming qualities, stinging nettle, which has anti-inflammatory qualities, and green tea, which is high in antioxidants and may help reduce inflammation.

Even if these herbs seem promising, people should always speak with a doctor before adding any new herbs to their regimen for managing their arthritis, particularly if they are already taking other medications.

Herbal treatments provide an all-natural and perhaps successful way to control flare-ups of arthritis.

Herbal supplements should be used carefully and under the supervision of healthcare professionals, as individual reactions to herbs can differ.

Overall arthritis management can be improved by using these herbs in a holistic strategy that may also include traditional medications and lifestyle changes.

CHAPTER THREE

ARTHRITIS TEA WITH HERBS

For many people, arthritis is a common ailment that causes inflammation in the joints and can be a source of ongoing discomfort. Even though there are many traditional medical therapies available, some people choose to manage their arthritis symptoms using alternative methods, such as herbal remedies. Particularly herbal teas have grown in popularity because of their ability to reduce inflammation and offer solace during flare-ups of arthritis.

Nettle Tea: A Brew Rich In Nutrients

The leaves of the stinging nettle plant are used to make nettle tea, which is well known for being high in nutrients. Antioxidants, vitamins, and minerals included in this herbal infusion may help lessen arthritis-related inflammation. Furthermore, nettle tea is thought to possess analgesic qualities, which may provide alleviation from arthritis-related discomfort. Nettle tea may help maintain joint health and lessen the effects of arthritis flare-ups when consumed regularly.

Green Tea: A Supercharged Antioxidant

A mainstay of traditional medicine, green tea is renowned for its strong antioxidant qualities. Green tea's polyphenols, especially epigallocatechin gallate (EGCG), have anti-inflammatory properties that may help people with arthritis. By aiding in the body's defense against free radicals, these antioxidants may help lessen joint inflammation. Including green tea in your daily routine could be a tasty and all-natural approach to promote joint health and reduce the symptoms of arthritis.

Tea with Chamomile: Reducing Inflammation

The chamomile plant yields chamomile tea, which is well known for its relaxing and anti-inflammatory qualities. The bioactive ingredients in chamomile, like chamazulene, may be able to reduce arthritis-related inflammation. In addition, chamomile tea has a reputation for being calming, which makes it advantageous for people with arthritis-related stress and strain. Drinking chamomile tea regularly may help promote relaxation and possibly assist in controlling flare-ups of arthritis.

Turmeric Tea: A Beneficial Drink

Curcumin, a substance with strong anti-inflammatory and antioxidant qualities, is found in turmeric, a vivid golden spice with a long history in traditional medicine.

A common option for people looking for all-natural arthritis treatments is turmeric tea, which is prepared by steeping turmeric in hot water.

Because curcumin modulates inflammatory pathways, it may be able to relieve arthritis-related joint pain and swelling. Adding turmeric tea to one's daily routine could be a tasty and healthful way to control the symptoms of arthritis.

In summary, herbal teas offer a viable option for anyone looking for all-natural ways to control flare-ups of their arthritis.

Turmeric tea, chamomile tea, green tea, and nettle tea each have special qualities that might help with pain relief, inflammation reduction, and joint health in general.

Although these herbal therapies can be used as part of a comprehensive strategy for managing arthritis, people should speak with healthcare providers before making big changes to their treatment regimens. As with any medical disease, treating the complexity of arthritis requires individualized, all-encompassing treatment.

CHAPTER FOUR

ESSENTIAL OLIVE OILS HEALTH

For many people, arthritis is a chronic and crippling sickness that is marked by inflammation and pain in the joints. Even while there are conventional treatments accessible, there is a growing interest in investigating alternative medicines, such as essential oil therapy. For millennia, people have prized these organic plant extracts for their medicinal qualities.

Lavender Oil: A Muscle-Relaxing Agent

Many people know that lavender oil has calming and relaxing effects. It can be especially helpful for reducing muscle tension and fostering calmness in the context of arthritis. Lavender oil has anti-inflammatory and analgesic qualities that make it a useful supplement for managing arthritis. Applying diluted lavender oil to the afflicted areas might help reduce stiffness in the muscles and promote relaxation in general.

Using Eucalyptus Oil To Reduce Joint Pain

It's common knowledge that eucalyptus oil can reduce joint pain and increase range of motion. People who are having flare-ups of their arthritis may get relief from its anti-inflammatory and analgesic properties. After diluting eucalyptus oil with a carrier oil, it can be applied topically to the afflicted joints. Furthermore, breathing in the eucalyptus oil-infused steam may have respiratory advantages, enhancing arthritis patients' general well-being.

Peppermint Oil: Reducing Heat

Because of its cooling effect, peppermint oil is a great option for reducing arthritis-related inflammation. Because of its analgesic and anti-inflammatory qualities, the menthol found in peppermint oil helps to reduce pain and swelling. Pain from arthritis can be relieved by applying diluted peppermint oil to the afflicted areas, which will feel cool and pleasant.

How To Safely Use Essential Oils

Essential oils can be quite helpful in managing arthritis, but it's important to use them carefully to prevent negative side effects. To make sure there are no allergies or sensitivities, a patch test should be done before using any essential oils.

To avoid irritating your skin, dilute essential oils with a carrier oil before using them. One common treatment for arthritis is to gently massage diluted oil into the afflicted joints. It can also be beneficial to inhale through techniques like steam inhalation or diffuser use.

When used in conjunction with a comprehensive management strategy, essential oils can alleviate symptoms and improve the general health of those with arthritis.

Those looking for natural alternatives have a variety of options thanks to the muscle-relaxing benefits of lavender oil, the joint pain alleviation of eucalyptus oil, and the inflammation-cooling effects of peppermint oil. However, to completely benefit from these essential oils in the context of arthritic flare-ups, safety must come first by using the recommended dilution and application techniques.

Dietary Suggestions

Flare-ups from arthritis can be difficult to control, but making some dietary adjustments can be very helpful in reducing symptoms and improving joint health in general. Concentrating on anti-inflammatory foods is a crucial part of adopting nutrition to manage arthritis. These foods are well-known for their capacity to lower bodily inflammation, which frequently contributes to flare-ups of arthritis.

Foods That Reduce Inflammation

Some foods have been shown to have anti-inflammatory qualities, which means that people who get flare-ups from their arthritis may benefit from consuming them. Omega-3 fatty acids, which are abundant in fatty fish like salmon, mackerel, and sardines, have strong anti-inflammatory properties. Furthermore, adding walnuts, chia seeds, and flaxseeds to the diet can offer a plant-based source of omega-3 fatty acids.

Vibrant fruits and vegetables are another type of diet that reduces inflammation. Broccoli, spinach, kale, cherries, and berries are full of phytochemicals and antioxidants that reduce inflammation. Vibrantly colored produce has ingredients that could improve joint health and lessen the intensity of arthritic symptoms.

Due to their well-known anti-inflammatory qualities, ginger and turmeric can both be beneficial additions to a diet meant to help manage arthritis. To reap the advantages of these spices, you can drink them as tea or add them to meals. Furthermore, green tea has been linked to anti-inflammatory properties that may help to lessen the symptoms of arthritis due to its high polyphenol content.

Items To Steer Clear Of

Eating anti-inflammatory foods is vital, but so is avoiding foods that worsen inflammation and cause flare-ups of arthritis. Processed foods can aggravate inflammation since they are heavy in harmful fats and processed sugars. Limiting the intake of dairy products and red meat, as these foods are known to cause inflammation, may also be advantageous.

Solanine is a substance found in nightshade vegetables including tomatoes, eggplants, and peppers that some people think may be linked to inflammation. Some people with arthritis decide to restrict their nightshades to see whether it helps with their symptoms, but more research is required to make a definitive connection.

The Value Of Hydration

The importance of staying hydrated in the context of managing arthritis cannot be emphasized. Water is vital for general health, and keeping the right amount of moisture in the body is critical for joint health. People with arthritis must make sure they are getting enough water throughout the day since dehydration can exacerbate the symptoms of arthritis.

Maintaining adequate hydration facilitates more fluid movement in the joints and lessens friction, which can cause discomfort and inflammation.

Water also helps the body flush out impurities, which creates a more hygienic environment inside. Drinking less sugary and caffeinated beverages and choosing water as your main beverage might be a healthy nutritional decision for people with arthritis.

The key to controlling arthritic flare-ups with diet is to eat a diet high in anti-inflammatory foods, be aware of potential triggers, and be properly hydrated.

As with any adjustments about health, seeking advice from a licensed dietitian or healthcare provider can offer tailored recommendations based on unique requirements and situations.

CHAPTER FIVE

CHANGES IN LIFESTYLE FOR THE MANAGEMENT OF ARTHRITIS

The inflammation of the joints that is associated with arthritis can have a serious effect on a person's quality of life. While lifestyle modifications can help reduce symptoms and avoid flare-ups, medicinal interventions are still an important part of controlling arthritis.

Workout And Extending

Stretching and regular exercise are crucial parts of an arthritis treatment program. Low-impact exercises that maintain joint flexibility and lessen stiffness include walking, cycling, and swimming. Exercises that stretch the muscles around afflicted joints can reduce stress and increase the range of motion. Strength training can also improve muscle support, which lessens the strain on the joints.

For those with arthritis, adding exercise to the daily schedule could be difficult at first, but there are several advantages to begin with mild activities and work your way up to more strenuous ones. A physical therapist or other healthcare provider should be consulted to develop a customized fitness program that takes into account each person's demands and limits.

Techniques For Stress Management

It is well known that stress aggravates the symptoms of arthritis, making the pain and discomfort worse. By using stress-reduction strategies, arthritis can be better managed and flare-ups can be avoided. Techniques like mindfulness, meditation, and deep breathing can help reduce tension and encourage relaxation.

Effective stress management requires locating and resolving the sources of stress in one's life. This could entail altering one's way of life, establishing reasonable objectives, and developing work prioritization skills. Counseling programs, support groups, and mental health specialists can all be helpful for those who are experiencing stress because of their arthritis.

Hygiene Of Sleep

Good sleep is essential for general health and well-being, and it's especially critical for people with arthritis. Insufficient sleep has the potential to cause flare-ups of arthritis by elevating inflammation and pain sensitivity. Developing healthy sleep hygiene habits can improve the quality of your sleep, which will lessen the symptoms of arthritis.

Good sleep hygiene includes establishing a cozy sleeping environment, sticking to a regular sleep schedule, and avoiding stimulants like caffeine right before bed. Purchasing pillows and a supportive mattress can also help to improve joint alignment and lessen discomfort when you sleep.

In conclusion, for those looking to reduce flare-ups and enhance their general well-being, implementing a comprehensive approach to arthritis care that incorporates lifestyle modifications is critical.

A more thorough and successful arthritis treatment plan may be achieved by adding regular exercise, stress reduction strategies, and a high priority on restful sleep.

CHAPTER SIX

HERBAL CURES FOR PARTICULAR CATEGORIES OF ARTHRITIS

For many people, arthritis is a prevalent inflammatory disease that affects the joints and causes persistent pain and suffering. Herbal therapies have acquired appeal due to their potential in treating arthritis symptoms, especially during flare-ups, despite the existence of conventional medications. In this talk, we'll look at a variety of herbal treatments designed to treat different kinds of arthritis, such as gout, rheumatoid arthritis, and osteoarthritis.

Arthritis In The Bones

The most common type of arthritis is called osteoarthritis, which is defined by the slow deterioration of joint cartilage and the underlying bone. The goals of herbal treatments for osteoarthritis are to lessen discomfort, lessen inflammation, and increase joint flexibility. Turmeric is well known for its anti-inflammatory qualities because it contains the active ingredient curcumin. By inhibiting inflammatory pathways, taking supplements containing turmeric or its derivatives may help manage the symptoms of osteoarthritis.

Ginger is another herb that's frequently used to treat osteoarthritis. Ginger's anti-inflammatory and antioxidant properties have shown promise in lowering pain and enhancing joint function. You can take ginger as a supplement, drink it as a tea, or add it to food. Furthermore, research has been done on the possibility that the anti-inflammatory herb Boswellia serrata can lessen the symptoms of osteoarthritis. Supplemental boswellia may improve joint function and suppress inflammatory chemicals.

The Rheumatoid Joint

An autoimmune disease called rheumatoid arthritis is typified by synovial inflammation, which causes swelling, stiffness, and discomfort in the joints. The main goals of herbal treatments for rheumatoid arthritis are frequently to lower inflammation and alter the immune system. Again, because of its anti-inflammatory and immunomodulatory qualities, turmeric helps to manage rheumatoid arthritis.

Green tea is another plant that may help with rheumatoid arthritis. Green tea, which is high in antioxidants and polyphenols, may help lower inflammation and delay the onset of joint injury. People with rheumatoid arthritis may find comfort by adding green tea to their daily diet or by taking green tea supplements.

Gout

Gout is a type of arthritis that is distinguished by the buildup of crystals of uric acid in the joints. Herbal treatments for gout frequently aim to lower inflammation and uric acid levels. The plant devil's claw, which has anti-inflammatory qualities, has long been used to treat gout symptoms. Supplements containing devil's claw may help lessen the discomfort and swelling brought on by gout episodes.

Another herbal medicine that has demonstrated promise in the management of gout is cherry extract. Certain substances found in cherries may reduce uric acid levels and reduce inflammation. For those with gout flare-ups, drinking cherry juice or taking pills containing cherry extract may help.

Herbal therapies offer a natural and comprehensive approach to managing arthritis symptoms, making them useful supplements to traditional treatments. Before including herbal therapies in their arthritis management strategy, people should speak with healthcare specialists because there may be interactions with drugs and individual reactions may differ.

CHAPTER SEVEN

HERBAL DOSES AND PREPARATIONS

Herbal remedies are available in a variety of forms, and each has special advantages for relieving arthritis. The next sections offer insights into the variety of herbal medicines accessible, ranging from tinctures and extracts to infusions and decoctions.

Herbal Decoctions And Infusions

In herbal infusions, the medicinal qualities of the plants are extracted by steeping them in hot water. Popular options for reducing arthritic symptoms include green tea, ginger, and turmeric. You can take these infusions daily to assist in easing pain and reduce inflammation. Furthermore, intense comfort is provided by decoctions, which are made by boiling herbs to extract their therapeutic ingredients. Due to their anti-inflammatory qualities, herbs like Boswellia and white willow bark are frequently employed in decoctions.

Extracts And Tinctures

Strong herbal preparations such as tinctures and extracts might be very helpful when arthritis flares up. plants are steeped in vinegar or alcohol to make tinctures, whereas extracts concentrate the components in plants using a solvent.

Herbs with anti-inflammatory and analgesic qualities that are frequently utilized in tinctures and extracts include comfrey, arnica, and devil's claw. To guarantee safety and effectiveness when utilizing these concentrated versions, proper dosage and administration are essential.

Guidelines For Dosage

The effectiveness of herbal treatments in treating arthritis symptoms depends on figuring out the right dose. Depending on the particular herb, the person's weight, and the intensity of the flare-up, the dosage may change. To establish customized dosage guidelines, speaking with a licensed herbalist or healthcare provider is advised. Following the suggested dosages is essential to minimize possible adverse effects and maximize the therapeutic advantages of herbal treatments.

Herbal treatments offer a comprehensive and all-natural means of easing the pain brought on by flare-ups of arthritis.

Herbal tinctures, extracts, decoctions, and infusions provide a variety of choices for people looking for non-traditional ways to relieve their symptoms. For herbal medicines to be safely and effectively included in arthritis management regimens, caution must be taken, prescribed dosages must be followed, and medical advice must be sought.

CHAPTER EIGHT

SAFETY MEASUREMENTS AND CONTACTS

Those with arthritis who are considering herbal remedies should put safety first and be mindful of any possible interactions. These treatments might be helpful, but there's a chance they could cause problems as well, particularly if taken with other drugs or in certain situations.

Speaking With A Medical Expert

Speak with a healthcare provider before adding herbal therapies to a regimen for managing arthritis.

A licensed healthcare professional can evaluate a patient's unique medical history, current medications, and possible drug interactions to provide tailored advice regarding the suitability of herbal remedies.

Medications And Possible Interactions

Certain herbal therapies may interfere with pharmaceuticals regularly used for arthritis. For example, turmeric and ginger may have blood-thinning characteristics, potentially enhancing the effects of anticoagulant drugs. Understanding these interactions is vital to avoid adverse effects and ensure the safe coexistence of herbal remedies and prescribed drugs.

Side Effects And Allergies

Individuals considering herbal remedies for arthritis should be vigilant about possible side effects and allergies.

Even though these remedies are natural, they can still induce adverse reactions in some individuals. Monitoring for symptoms such as allergic reactions, gastrointestinal issues, or changes in blood pressure is essential to address any potential complications promptly.

while herbal remedies may offer a natural approach to managing arthritis flare-ups, a cautious and informed approach is paramount. Safety precautions, consultation with healthcare professionals, and awareness of potential interactions and side effects are essential components of integrating herbal remedies into an arthritis management plan.

CHAPTER NINE

SUCCESS STORIES

Arthritis, a condition characterized by inflammation of the joints, can be debilitating and affect one's quality of life. Many individuals have explored alternative approaches, such as herbal remedies, to manage arthritis flare-ups successfully. Success stories serve as anecdotal evidence of the effectiveness of these remedies in providing relief and improving overall well-being.

Personal Testimonials

Individuals who have experienced arthritis flare-ups often share personal testimonials detailing their journey with herbal remedies. These narratives offer insights into the specific herbs, formulations, and lifestyle changes that have played a crucial role in managing their symptoms. Personal testimonials provide a firsthand account of the challenges faced and the positive outcomes achieved through the integration of herbal remedies into their arthritis management regimen.

Case Studies

In-depth case studies delve into specific instances where individuals have employed herbal remedies to address arthritis flare-ups. These studies often examine the background of the individuals, the severity of their arthritis, and the herbal interventions implemented. Case studies contribute valuable information about the efficacy, safety, and potential challenges associated with using herbal remedies for arthritis management.

Herbal remedies encompass a wide range of natural substances derived from plants, each with its unique properties and potential benefits for arthritis sufferers. From traditional remedies passed down through generations to contemporary herbal supplements, individuals explore various options to find relief from arthritis symptoms.

Understanding Arthritis Flare-Ups

Arthritis flare-ups are characterized by increased inflammation, pain, and stiffness in the joints. These episodes can be triggered by factors such as stress, changes in weather, physical activity, or underlying health conditions. Herbal remedies aim to address these flare-ups by targeting inflammation, improving joint mobility, and enhancing overall joint health.

Common Herbal Remedies For Arthritis Flare-Ups

Turmeric and Curcumin: Known for its anti-inflammatory properties, turmeric and its active compound, curcumin, have shown promise in reducing arthritis-related inflammation and pain. These can be consumed as a spice in food or taken as supplements.

Ginger: Ginger has anti-inflammatory and antioxidant effects that may help alleviate arthritis symptoms. It can be consumed in various forms, including fresh ginger in meals, ginger tea, or as a supplement.

Boswellia: Derived from the resin of the Boswellia tree, Boswellia extract has anti-inflammatory properties and may aid in reducing arthritis-related swelling and discomfort.

Willow Bark: Willow bark contains salicin, a compound similar to aspirin, which may help alleviate pain and inflammation associated with arthritis. It is available in supplement form.

Devil's Claw: This herb contains anti-inflammatory qualities and may be used to alleviate arthritis pain and enhance joint function. Devil's Claw can be taken as a supplement.

Fish Oil: Rich in omega-3 fatty acids, fish oil has anti-inflammatory effects and may help relieve joint discomfort and stiffness. It is often provided as a supplement.

Implementing Herbal Remedies Safely

While herbal medicines might offer relief for arthritis flare-ups, it is crucial to approach their use with caution. Consulting with a healthcare practitioner before introducing herbal supplements into one's routine is important, as some herbs may interact with drugs or have contraindications for certain health problems.

success stories, personal testimonials, and case studies collectively illustrate the positive influence of herbal treatments on controlling arthritic flare-ups. As individuals continue to explore alternate techniques, these accounts give significant insights into the varied strategies adopted to increase the quality of life for persons coping with arthritis.

CONCLUSION

herbal remedies offer a natural and potentially successful alternative to controlling arthritic flare-ups. While some therapies show potential, patients with arthritis need to contact healthcare specialists before adopting them into their treatment programs. The route to controlling arthritis is multidimensional, needing a holistic approach that tackles triggers, lifestyle variables, and the integration of both conventional and natural therapies.

Recap Of Herbal Remedies

In this investigation of herbal therapies for arthritic flare-ups, we reviewed the potential advantages of turmeric, ginger, Boswellia, willow bark, stinging nettle, and cat's claw. Each of these herbs contains unique qualities that may contribute to relieving inflammation and pain associated with arthritis. It is crucial to approach herbal treatments with an understanding of their mechanisms and potential interactions with other medications.

Motivation For The Upcoming Trip

Although treating flare-ups can be difficult when one has arthritis, adopting a holistic approach that incorporates herbal medicines can help. Maintaining awareness, collaborating closely with medical specialists, and modifying one's lifestyle to support general health is crucial. People can travel the path ahead with a stronger sense of empowerment and control over their arthritic symptoms by combining conventional and herbal approaches.